NATURAL HEALING WITH DMSO.

Healing Guide With Dimethyl Sulfoxide (Dmso) For Treating Bladder Pain, Arthritis, Rheumatoid Arthritis, Trigeminal Neuralgia (TN), and Scleroderma.

By

Charles Amelia.

Table of Contents

CHAPTER ONE...6

CONCEPT OF DMSO...6

Dimethyl Sulfoxide (DMSO)..7

What Is DMSO? 7

CHAPTER TWO...9

DISCOVERY AND HISTORY OF DMSO.................................9

Chemical Build Of DMSO. 11

Chemical And Physical Properties Of The DMSO. 12

CHAPTER THREE. 14

MEDICAL AND PHARMACEUTICAL APPLICATION..................14

Interstitial Cystitis/Bladder..14

Some Common Symptoms And Signs...............................15

Major Causes Of Interstitial Cystitis. 16

Risk Factors Associated With Interstitial Cystitis. 16

Interstitial Cystitis/Bladder Using DMSO as A Treatment ...18

Addition Of Cryoprotectant: 19

CHAPTER FOUR...21

ARTHRITIS..21

The Concept Of Rheumatoid Arthritis And The Application
Of DMSO..21

Common Symptoms Of Rheumatoid Arthritis. 22

Major causes of Rheumatoid arthritis(RA?).......................23

Menace Factor For Rheumatoid Arthritis............................23

Features That Increase Risk. 23

Treatment Of Rheumatoid Arthritis. 25

How To Manage Your Rheumatoid Arthritis And Improve Healthy Quality Of Life. 28

Application Of DMSO In Treating Rheumatoid Arthritis......28

Precaution In Using DMSO For Rheumatoid Arthritis.........29

CHAPTER FIVE 31

TRIGEMINAL NEURALGIA (TIC DOULOUREUX). 31

Symptom's Of TN. 31

Trigeminal Nerves. 32

People Likely To Get Trigeminal Neuralgia. 34

Causes Of Trigeminal Neuralgia (TN)...............................35

Pains Of Trigeminal Neuralgia. 36

Diagnosis Of Trigeminal Neuralgias................................37

Treatment Of Trigeminal Neuralgia................................38

Medications For Trigeminal Neuralgia. 39

Trigeminal Nerve Block. 40

Trigeminal Neuralgia Surgery. 40

Rhizotomy Techniques..42

Microvascular Decompression.......................................44

Additional Treatments. 45

Application Of DMSO in Treating Trigeminal Neuralgia. 46

CHAPTER SIX 47

SCLERODERMA. 47

    What is Scleroderma: 47

    Kinds Of Scleroderma. 47

    Causes of Scleroderma. 49

    Risk factor of Scleroderma. 49

    Scleroderma Symptoms. 50

    Diagnosis Of Scleroderma. 50

    Scleroderma Complications. 51

    Scleroderma Treatment. 51

    DMSO Application In Treating Scleroderma. 52

    Precaution In Using DMSO For Scleroderma. ...53

CHAPTER SEVEN. 54

Uses And Effectiveness. 54

    Effective On: 54

    Most Effective On: 54

    Some Ineffectiveness: 55

    Cancer 55

Other Uses of DMSO Based on Research. 56

    Side Effects In Using DMSO. 58

    Safety Special Precautions. 59

    General Dosing. 60

    Application To The Skin. 60

Inside The Bladder. 61

CHAPTER ONE.

CONCEPT OF DMSO.

Dimethyl sulfoxide (DMSO) is one of the most commonly used drugs in life sciences.

In addition to its use as a valuable Cryoprotectant, DMSO is considered by many to be a versatile solvent that can efficiently dissolve both polar and non-polar compounds.

For this reason, numerous studies have been conducted investigating the different therapeutic properties of different compounds and extracts dissolved in DMSO.

It is an odourless and transparent substance with amazing properties.

Think of it as a multipurpose assistant in our environment

Other studies have directly investigated the modulatory effects of DMSO in specific pathological conditions.

Dimethyl Sulfoxide (DMSO).

What Is DMSO?

Dimethyl sulfoxide (DMSO) is a chemical that dissolves many organic and inorganic substances.

DMSO is Available as a prescription drug and dietary supplement.

DMSO helps drugs pass through the skin and can affect proteins, carbohydrates, fats, and water in the body.

DMSO is used for bladder infections (interstitial cystitis), body pain that usually occurs after an injury, and leakage of intravenous drugs from veins into surrounding skin and tissues.

It is also used for osteoarthritis, bedsores, stomach ulcers, and many other conditions, although there is not enough scientific evidence for most of these other uses.

DMSO can be injected intravenously, topically, or orally in certain situations to reduce cystitis and associated pain. In some cases, it is used with prescription drugs to improve their ability to penetrate the skin and enter the bloodstream.

<u>CHAPTER TWO.</u>

<u>DISCOVERY AND HISTORY OF DMSO.</u>

Dimethyl sulfoxide (DMSO) is a widely used solvent that is miscible with water and many

organic solvents. It has several names, including methyl sulfoxide, sulfinylbismethane, and dozens of trade names.

DMSO is a laboratory and industrial solvent for many gases, synthetic fibres, dyes, hydrocarbons, salts and natural products. Because it is aprotic, relatively inert, nontoxic, and stable at high temperatures, it is a commonly used solvent in chemical reactions.

In the 1960s, scientists discovered that DMSO penetrates human skin with little effect on tissue; and the solvent has been tested as a way to deliver drugs into the body as an alternative to oral dosage forms or injections. Since then, DMSO has been used in several transdermal drug delivery systems (ie, patches).

In 1978, the US Food and Drug Administration approved its use to relieve the symptoms of chronic interstitial cystitis (bladder pain syndrome), the only FDA approval of DMSO as an actual medication.

As you might expect in the 1960s, DMSO was tested as an alternative medicine to reduce inflammation and as a solvent for injecting illegal drugs like cocaine.

It has also been falsely advertised as an anti-cancer cure. In 1965, the FDA shut down much of that activity, banning clinical trials with DMSO because the compound changed the refractive index of the lenses of the test animals' eyes. The ban was lifted in 1980 when intense interest in the substance declined.

Researchers are still looking at DMSO as a potential drug treatment. In 2016, Gerald Krystal and colleagues from the British Columbia Cancer Agency (Vancouver), the University of British Columbia (Vancouver) and Vancouver General Hospital reported that DMSO inhibits the production of inflammatory cytokines by human blood cells, thus reducing autoimmune arthritis. The authors also investigated whether DMSO has anticancer effects; they concluded that they could not confirm that this was the case.

<u>Chemical Build Of DMSO.</u>

The DMSO is mainly soluble in water and it has a wide solubility with various organic solvents among others not mentioned. Researchers and many other users address or call the DMSO other names such as sulfinyl methane, methyl sulfoxide and many more brand names.

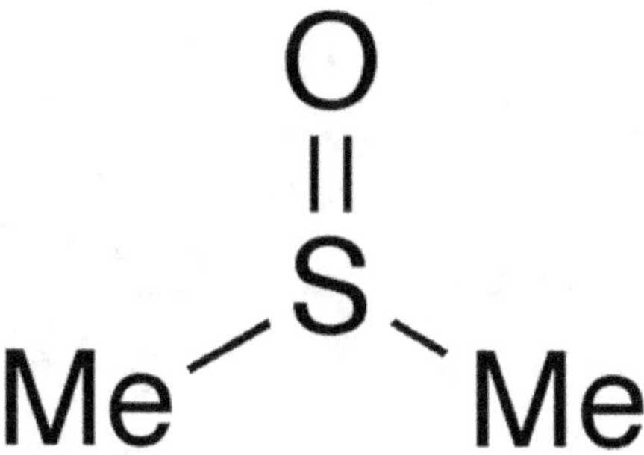

Fig 1.1

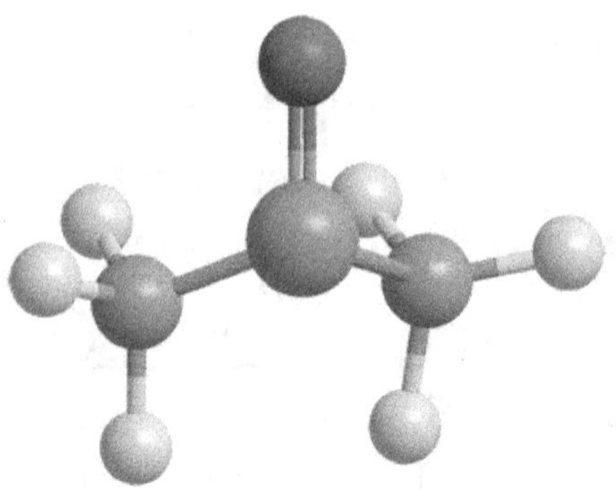

Fig 1.2

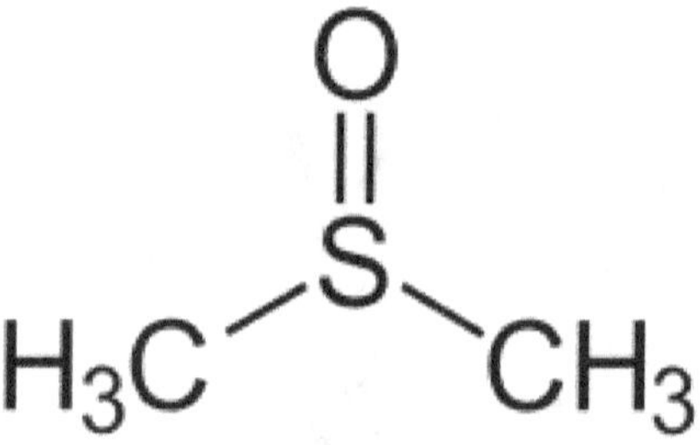

$$\overset{\displaystyle O}{\underset{\displaystyle H_3C \qquad CH_3}{\|\;\;S}}$$

Fig 1.3

<u>**Chemical And Physical Properties Of The DMSO.**</u>

Briefly, other facts have it that the DMSO has an empirical formula C_2H_6OS with a relative molecular mass of about 78.13 g/mol, and it's a colorless substance with an insignificant cabbage or garlic odor. And have a boiling point of 189^0c and a melting point of 19^0c, and is soluble in water

CHAPTER THREE.

MEDICAL AND PHARMACEUTICAL APPLICATION.

Dimethyl sulfoxide (DMSO) is primarily used to relieve pain and promote the healing of wounds, burns, and musculoskeletal injuries. Dimethyl sulfoxide (DMSO) is also used topically to treat other severe or unpleasant painful conditions such as headache, inflammation, osteoarthritis, rheumatoid arthritis, and severe facial pain called tic douloureux.

Interstitial Cystitis/Bladder.

The fact that the urinary system makes up the kidneys, ureters and bladders hence, When you have interstitial cystitis, the bladder walls become irritated and inflamed (pictured right) compared to the walls of a normal bladder. With interstitial cystitis, these signals are mixed - you feel the urge to urinate more often and with less urine than most people.

Interstitial cystitis most commonly affects women and can have a long-term impact on quality of life. The interstitial may at this moment have no

14

potential cure but can be managed with some medications and with the DMSO application to reduce pains in users.

<u>Some Common Symptoms And Signs.</u>

Different people's contact with interstitial cystitis has different symptoms and signs. With interstitial cystitis, symptoms change over time and may occur intermittently in response to common triggers such as menstruation, prolonged sitting, stress, exercise, and sexual activity.

Symptoms may include the following:

- Pain between the female pelvis or vagina and anus
- Experience Pain between the man's scrotum and anus as it may.
- Chronic pelvic pain
- Painful sensation during sex
- Urgent need to urinate

The severity of symptoms varies from person to person, and some people may experience symptom-free periods. Meanwhile, the signs and symptoms of interstitial cystitis may look like those of a severe urinary tract infection, there is usually no trace of infection. Symptoms may be more severe if a person is currently managing or getting urinary tract infections.

<u>Major Causes Of Interstitial Cystitis.</u>

The exact cause of interstitial cystitis is unknown, but many factors can contribute. For example, people with interstitial cystitis may also have damage to the lining (epithelium) of the bladder. Epithelial leakage may allow toxic substances in the urine to irritate the bladder wall. There are some factors not proven though but can contribute to the cause of interstitial cystitis may include infection, autoimmune reaction, heredity, infection, and or allergy.

<u>Risk Factors Associated With Interstitial Cystitis.</u>

These risk factors include the following;

- **Your gender**: Women are diagnosed with interstitial cystitis more often than men. Symptoms in men can mimic interstitial cystitis, but they are more often associated with prostatitis.

- your age: Most people with interstitial cystitis are diagnosed in their 30s.
- Chronic pain disorder: Interstitial cystitis may be associated with other chronic pain disorders such as irritable bowel syndrome or fibromyalgia.
Some complications that can result from interstitial cystitis. Interstitial cystitis can cause several complications, including:
- Decreased bladder capacity: Interstitial cystitis can cause a stiffening of the bladder wall, which allows the bladder to urinate less.
- Worse quality of life: frequent urination and pain can interfere with social activities, work and other daily activities.
- Problems with sexual intimacy: Frequent urination and pain can strain your personal relationships and sexual intimacy can suffer.

Interstitial Cystitis/Bladder Using DMSO as A Treatment.

Bladder pain and/or the need to urinate are symptoms of a condition called (IC/BPS) which is interstitial cystitis/bladder pain syndrome. Because the aetiology of IC/BPS is unknown, treatment decisions are primarily based on physician and personal preference rather than research findings.

The FDA which is the Food and Drug Administration a body in charge, has approved liquid dimethyl sulfoxide (DMSO) for the treatment of interstitial cystitis and bladder pain syndrome (IC/BPS). DMSO should be inserted into the bladder with a temporary catheter and left in place for at least 20 minutes.

The entire treatment may take up to six weeks or thereabout in administering the DMSO daily to patients and so may still feel pains for a while before their healing process begins.

Other Bladder Infusions: To reduce discomfort, some physicians recommend mixing drugs introduced into the bladder through a catheter.

This can be done in a doctor's office or you can learn how to care for yourself at home.

Addition Of Cryoprotectant:

Dimethyl sulfoxide (DMSO) is currently the most commonly used cryoprotectant for cryopreservation of hematopoietic stem cells. DMSO is a versatile solvent or agent that can equilibrate cell membranes under rapidly changing conditions and prevent the formation of intracellular ice crystals during freezing and the release of heat during phase changes. DMSO has been reported to be toxic to stem cells at room temperature.

Therefore, the researchers emphasize the findings that it must be added to the cells before controlled freezing to 4°C and immediate cryopreservation.

A final concentration of 10% DMSO with albumin or human serum is typical. Some centres use hydroxyethyl starch to stabilize cell membranes and reduce the amount of DMSO to 5%.

 A new cryopreservation agent, (Bio Life Solutions Inc., Corning, NY), is also readily available. This compound modulates cell biochemistry during freezing and does not contain serum, proteins or DMSO.

CHAPTER FOUR

ARTHRITIS.

The concept of arthritis has to do with the tenderness and swelling of the joints affected. The main symptoms of arthritis are joint pain and stiffness, which commonly get worse with age.

Osteoarthritis and rheumatoid arthritis are the two well-known types of arthritis. We will look at Rheumatoid arthritis as a key study and how DMSO can be used or applied to reduce pains

The Concept Of Rheumatoid Arthritis And The Application Of DMSO.

Rheumatoid arthritis, or RA, is an autoimmune disease. This means that the immune system mistakenly attacks the body's healthy cells, causing inflammation (painful swelling) in the affected body area.

Rheumatoid arthritis primarily affects the joints, usually multiple joints at the same time.

Rheumatoid arthritis often affects the joints of the hands, wrists, and knees.

In joints with rheumatoid arthritis, the lining of the joint becomes inflamed, leading to joint tissue damage.

Common Symptoms Of Rheumatoid Arthritis.

Rheumatoid arthritis has periods when symptoms get worse, called exacerbations and times when symptoms get better, called remissions.

Symptoms and signs of rheumatoid arthritis include:

- Stiffness in more than one joint
- Pain or aching in more than one joint
- Stiffness in more than one joint
- Tenderness and swelling in more than one joint
- Both sides of the body encounter the same symptoms such as both arms and legs. Weakness
- Fever

♦ Fatigue or tiredness Weight loss and others

Major causes of Rheumatoid arthritis(RA?).

RA is the result of immune reactions in which the body's immune system attacks its healthy cells.

Although the specific cause of rheumatoid arthritis is unknown, several factors may increase your risk of developing rheumatoid arthritis.

Menace Factor For Rheumatoid Arthritis.

Finders and researchers have investigated a variety of genetic and environmental factors to determine whether they alter a person's risk of developing rheumatoid arthritis.

Features That Increase Risk.

- Gender: New cases of rheumatoid arthritis usually occur two to three times more often in women than in men.
- Age: Rheumatoid arthritis can occur at any age, but the likelihood increases with age. RA disease most commonly occurs in adults in their 60s or thereabouts.

- **Hereditary:** People with certain genes have a higher risk of developing rheumatoid arthritis. These genes, called HLA class II (human leukocyte antigen) genotypes, can also make arthritis worse. People with these genes may have the highest risk of developing RA if they are exposed to environmental factors such as smoking or if they are obese.
- **Smoking**: Some studies show that smoking increases the risk of developing rheumatoid arthritis and can make the disease worse.

Conception or live birth: Women who have never given birth may be at increased risk of developing rheumatoid arthritis. How is rheumatoid arthritis diagnosed? Rheumatoid arthritis is diagnosed by checking your symptoms, doing a physical exam, and doing X-rays and lab tests. Diagnose rheumatoid arthritis early, within 6 months of symptoms, so people with rheumatoid arthritis can start treatment.. slow or stop the progression of the disease (such as joint damage) That's the best thing to do.

Diagnosis and effective treatment, especially those that suppress or control inflammation, can help reduce the harmful effects of rheumatoid arthritis.

<u>**Treatment Of Rheumatoid Arthritis.**</u>

Rheumatoid arthritis should be diagnosed and treated by a doctor or team of doctors who specialize in caring for patients with rheumatoid arthritis.

This is especially important because the signs and symptoms of rheumatoid arthritis are not specific and can resemble those of other inflammatory joint diseases.

A doctor who specializes in arthritis is called a rheumatologist and can make the correct diagnosis.

To find a provider near you, visit our external icon database of rheumatologists.

It's key to note that this type of arthritis (Rheumatoid arthritis) RA is majorly managed and treated with medications effectively if followed right prescription, other strategies or methods can be applied if well knowledgeable about RA.

Treatment of rheumatoid arthritis usually involves the use of drugs called disease-modifying anti-rheumatic drugs (DMARDs) that slow the progression of the disease and prevent joint deformities.

Biological response modifiers (biologics) are drugs that provide effective second-line treatment.

In addition to medications, rheumatoid arthritis can also be treated with self-management strategies that have been proven to reduce pain and disability and allow you to pursue activities that are important to you.

Rheumatoid arthritis patients can reduce pain and improve joint function by learning five simple and effective arthritis treatment strategies.

Major complication associated with Rheumatoid arthritis

Rheumatoid arthritis (RA) has many physical and social consequences that can affect quality of life.

It can cause pain, disability, and early death.

- **Early heart disease**: People with rheumatoid arthritis (RA) are also at increased risk of other chronic diseases, such as heart disease and diabetes. To prevent heart disease in patients with rheumatoid arthritis, the treatment of rheumatoid arthritis also focuses on reducing the risk factors for heart disease. For example, doctors recommend that patients with rheumatoid arthritis stop smoking and lose weight...
- Obesity: Overweight people with RA have a higher risk of heart disease risk factors such as high blood pressure and high cholesterol. Being overweight also increases the risk of chronic diseases such as heart disease and diabetes. Finally, obese RA patients benefit less from therapy than non-obese RA patients.

<u>**How To Manage Your Rheumatoid Arthritis And Improve Healthy Quality Of Life.**</u>

Rheumatoid arthritis affects many aspects of daily life, including work, leisure, and social activities. Fortunately, several cost-effective strategies have been proven to improve the quality of life in the community including the following:

- Reduce or stop smoking.
- Active physically.
- Maintain a healthy weight.

<u>**Application Of DMSO In Treating Rheumatoid Arthritis.**</u>

Studies have shown that topical application of DMSO reduces the production of inflammatory compounds such as cytokines in the joints and white blood cells of mice. It may be most effective at concentrations of 0.5% to 2%.

It effectively penetrates human skin and is an excellent solvent or carrier liquid for containing pharmacological compounds in topical treatments. DMSO is not yet approved by the **FDA** as a treatment for arthritis, but it has been shown to have anti-inflammatory properties and relieve joint pain.

Its safety and dosing continue to be studied in humans, and it may have potential as an alternative or supplement to common arthritis medications.

Therefore, experts continue to explore alternative treatments that effectively treat arthritis symptoms without negative side effects.

Dimethyl sulfoxide (DMSO) treatment may be one such alternative

25% DMSO gel has been used 3 times a day, and 45.5% DMSO topical solution has been applied 4 times a day.

Precaution In Using DMSO For Rheumatoid Arthritis.

DMSO is not currently approved by the FDA to treat arthritis.

Additionally, the effectiveness of DMSO is dose-dependent and is only effective over a narrow concentration range of 0.5% to 2%.

For example, DMSO has been shown to reduce the amount and function of white blood cells at high doses and may affect immune system function.

The most commonly reported symptoms were gastrointestinal and skin-related.

However, reactions were rare, mild, and short-lived.

However, at 0.05%, DMSO did not provide any benefit to rheumatoid arthritis patients, although no side effects were reported at lower doses.

Reported symptoms also vary depending on the route of administration.

Some people experienced skin reactions when administered topically, while experts observed mild effects on the cardiac system when administered intravenously.

CHAPTER FIVE

TRIGEMINAL NEURALGIA (TIC DOULOUREUX).

Trigeminal neuralgia (TN), (also known as tic douloureux,) is a type of severe pain disorder often caused by sudden, chronic pain in the face. It affects the trigeminal nerve, or the fifth cranial nerve, which transmits sensations and nerve signals to many parts of the head and face.

Trigeminal neuralgia (TN) is a type of neuropathic pain usually caused by nerve damage or injury.

Symptom's Of TN.

Basic symptoms include the following:

- Sudden, severe pain, usually on one side of the face.
- Pain attacks that can last from a few seconds to about two minutes.
- Numbness or tingling.
- A burning, throbbing, shock-like, or painful sensation.

• Regular pains for a few days or weeks even longer, constant pains every day.

<u>Trigeminal Nerves.</u>

The trigeminal nerves are a pair of cranial nerves that connect the brain and brainstem to different parts of the brain, the head, body and neck. All 12 nerves branch out to serve two sides of your body and brain.

Each nerve also has three branches that control sensation in the upper, middle and lower parts of the face.

• The ophthalmic or superior branch supplies sensation to most of the scalp, forehead and front of the head.

• The middle branch of the lower jaw stimulates the cheek, upper jaw, upper lip, teeth and gums, and the sides of the nose.

• Mandible, or lower jaw, supplies nerves to the lower jaw, teeth and gums, and the lower lip. The disorder can affect more than one branch of the nerve. In some rare cases, both sides of the face may be affected at different times or even less often at the same time (bilateral TN).

TN finds itself having two main types at the moment as listed below:

Type 1: This is the typical or "classic" form of disorder. It causes severe, intermittent, sudden, burning or shock-like pain in the face. The pain lasts from a few seconds to two minutes per episode.

These attacks can happen very close together, in episodes that can last up to two hours. Severe flashes of pain can be triggered by shaking or touching the cheek (such as shaving, washing your face or applying makeup), brushing your teeth, eating, drinking, talking or being exposed to the wind.

The pain may affect a small area of your face or spread. Pain attacks rarely occur during sleep. Due to the intensity of the pain, some people may avoid daily activities or social contact for fear of an imminent attack.

Type 2: Type 2 pains are usually less severe than those of type 1. It is majorly caused by frequent aching, and stabbing pains alike which create some typical forms of the disorder and discomfort.

 You can have both forms of trigeminal neuralgia, sometimes at the same time.

The pains are devastating and can be so physical and mental. TN attacks typically stop for some time and then return.

However, looking at other conditions or in some cases mentioned can be in increasing progress which signifies the attacks may be more severe over time, with lower or little pains attached before they come around again.

In progressive TN, the pain-free intervals eventually disappear and medication to control the pain becomes less effective.

<u>People Likely To Get Trigeminal Neuralgia.</u>

- A blood vessel that, leaving the brainstem, presses on the trigeminal nerve. This compression causes the protective layer (myelin sheath) around the nerve to wear down or become damaged.

- Multiple sclerosis, a disease that causes the trigeminal nerve and the myelin sheath to deteriorate
- Damage to the trigeminal nerve (perhaps from sinus surgery, oral surgery, stroke, or facial trauma)

Causes Of Trigeminal Neuralgia (TN).

The trigeminal neuralgia (TN) is mainly caused when the trigeminal nerves that are found at the base part of the brain undergo compression. In most cases, this is due to pressure on the nerve root.

A brain tumour can also compress the trigeminal nerve. Trigeminal neuralgia can develop as a result of ageing or be related to multiple sclerosis or a similar disease that damages the myelin sheath that protects certain nerves. Trigeminal neuralgia can also be caused by surgical wounds, stroke or facial injuries. Trigeminal neuralgia can run in families, possibly because family members have inherited abnormal blood vessel formation.

Multiple sclerosis or a tumour although rare can also cause trigeminal neuralgia. Researchers are investigating whether herpetic neuralgia (caused by shingles) may be related to the condition.

Pains Of Trigeminal Neuralgia.

The trigeminal nerve divides into three branches: ophthalmic, maxillary and mandibles. Each branch gives sensations to different areas of the face.

Depending on which branch and which part of the nerve is irritated, trigeminal neuralgia can be felt anywhere on the face. It is most often felt in the lower part of the face. The intensity of the pain is extraordinary: some people report that it is worse than a heart attack, the removal of kidney stones or even childbirth.

The onset of trigeminal neuralgia may begin with tingling or numbness in the face. The pain occurs in intermittent bursts that last from a few seconds to two minutes and increase until the pain is almost constant.

Surgeries can last a few weeks or months, followed by a pain-free period that can last a year or more. Although trigeminal pain may seem to go away, it always returns, often more intensely.

In some cases, instead of sharp stabbing pain, trigeminal neuralgia appears as a constant dull pain.

This and other variations in symptoms are sometimes described as "atypical trigeminal neuralgia."

Diagnosis Of Trigeminal Neuralgias.

The diagnosis of trigeminal neuralgia involves a physical examination and a detailed medical history to rule out other causes of facial pain. Your healthcare provider (usually a primary care physician or neurologist) will ask about the frequency and intensity of the pain, what seems to be causing it, and what makes it feel better or worse. Because there is no single test for trigeminal neuralgia, determining the nature of the pain is key to diagnosis.

Your provider may also recommend imaging or laboratory tests, such as a CAT scan of the trigeminal nerve and surrounding areas or a high-resolution MRI. These tests can help determine if the pain is due to a tumour blood vessel abnormality or undiagnosed multiple sclerosis. Some advanced MRI techniques can help the doctor see where a blood vessel is pressing on a branch of the trigeminal nerve.

If doctors suspect you have TN1, they may ask you to try a short course of anticonvulsants. If the drug helps, it helps support the diagnosis of TN1. Diagnosing TN2 is more complicated, but doctors may ask you to try low doses of tricyclic antidepressants (such as amitriptyline and nortriptyline) to see if it helps. If so, a positive answer supports the diagnosis of TN2.

Treatment Of Trigeminal Neuralgia.

Some medications like tablets or pills may not work for the treatment of some illnesses hence the doctor may request a suggestion such as medical surgery to help carry out the treatment.

Medications For Trigeminal Neuralgia.

These several method can help to treat TN

- Anticonvulsant drugs. Anticonvulsants are used to prevent nerve burn. They are usually effective in treating TN1, but often less effective in TN2. Medicine that may include topiramate, phenytoin, lamotrigine and valproic acid other medication may also include oxcarbamazepine.
- Antidepressants. Tricyclic antidepressants such as amitriptyline or nortriptyline can be used to relieve pain.   Common pain relievers (such as aspirin and ibuprofen) and opioid medications such as hydrocodone usually do not help with the sharp, recurring pain caused by TN1. However, some TN2 patients find opioids helpful.

However, many people with trigeminal neuralgia can manage the condition successfully with medication for years. Trigeminal neuralgia is treated with the same medications used to control seizures, including carbamazepine, gabapentin, and similar agents. Some medications may require regular blood tests to check your white blood cell count, platelet count, sodium level, and liver function.

Your neurologist or primary care physician can help you choose the best drug and the most appropriate dose. Most patients start with low doses and gradually increase

The dose is under clinical supervision until the best pain relief and the fewest side effects are achieved.

Trigeminal Nerve Block.

Nerve injections are injections (with a steroid drug or other substance) into different parts of a nerve to reduce pain. They can provide temporary pain relief for people with trigeminal neuralgia. Several injections are usually required to achieve the desired relief, and the effect may last for different people for different periods.

Trigeminal Neuralgia Surgery.

If the medication does not relieve the pain or causes intolerable side effects such as cognitive impairment, memory loss, excessive fatigue, bone marrow failure or allergies, the doctor may recommend surgical treatment. Because TN can be a progressive disease that becomes resistant to drugs over time, people often seek surgical treatment. Treating TN have several methods among which is neurosurgical procedures.

The choice of procedure depends on the nature of the pain; your preferences, physical health, blood pressure and previous operations; the presence of multiple sclerosis and the distribution of trigeminal nerve involvement (especially if the superior/ophthalmic branch is involved).

You can expect some facial numbness after many of these procedures, and TN often returns even if the procedure was initially successful. Depending on the procedure, other risks of TN surgery include hearing loss, balance problems, cerebrospinal fluid (a fluid that washes the brain and spinal cord), infection, and pain anaesthesia (a type of nerve pain that causes both superficial numbness and deep numbness). burning pain) and (rarely) stroke.

Some procedures are performed on an outpatient basis, while others may involve more complex surgery that is performed under general anaesthesia and requires hospitalization.

<u>Rhizotomy Techniques.</u>

Rhizotomy (rhyolysis) is a procedure in which nerve fibres are damaged to prevent pain. Rhizotomy of TN always causes some sensory disturbances and facial numbness. Below are means outlined to treat trigeminal neuralgia using the rhizotomy format.

- Balloon compression uses the balloon tip of a small catheter that presses part of the trigeminal nerve against the hard edge of the covering of the brain (dura) and the skull. It damages the insulation of the nerves involved in the light touch of the face and can relieve trigeminal neuralgia. Pain relief from balloon compression usually lasts one to two years. Balloon compression is usually an outpatient procedure. It is performed in the operating room under general anaesthesia.

- When glycerol is injected, a drug is used to relieve pain that damages the insulation of the fibres of the trigeminal nerve. Injecting glycerol requires sedating the person with intravenous drugs. This is usually an outpatient procedure. Pain from glycerin injections usually lasts one to two years. The procedure can be repeated several times.

- Radiofrequency thermal injury (also known as "RF ablation" or "RF injury") uses heat to damage the pain-producing nerve fibres in the trigeminal nerve. In anaesthesia, a needle is placed near the trigeminal nerve and gradually heated with an electrode, which damages the nerve fibres. It may be necessary to reduce more than one procedure.

- Pain to an acceptable level while maintaining touch. Pain relief can be permanent, but about half of those treated this way have pain that returns within 3-4 years. These techniques are carried out on a prescribed method as recommended.

<u>Microvascular Decompression.</u>

Microvascular decompression (MVD) is the most invasive surgery for TN but offers the least likelihood of pain recurrence. This involves relieving pressure from surrounding blood vessels that either surround or touch the nerve.

A small opening is made through the skull and the surgeon places a soft pad between the nerve and the blood vessel (usually an artery) pressing on the nerve. Unlike a rhizotomy, the goal is not to numb the face after this surgery. MVD is an inpatient therapy performed under general anaesthesia. People usually stay in the hospital for several days after the procedure, and it usually takes several weeks to fully recover from the procedure. Pain is constant in about half of people with MVD. For others, the pain returns within 12 to 15 years.

A neurectomy (also called a partial neurectomy), which involves cutting part of the nerve, may be performed near the nerve's entry point in the brainstem during MVD if the surgeon finds that no blood vessels are pressing on the trigeminal nerve.

A neurectomy can also be performed by cutting the superficial branches of the trigeminal nerve of the face. A neurectomy causes long-term numbness in the face, which is acquired by the cut nerve or nerve branch. But the nerve can regrow and sensation can return over time. In connection with a neurectomy, there is a risk of painful anaesthesia.

Surgical treatment of TN2 is usually more problematic than TN1, especially if preoperative brain imaging does not show compression of the trigeminal vessels.

Many neurosurgeons do not recommend MVD or rhizotomy when TN2 symptoms predominate over TN1 unless vascular compression is confirmed. MVD for TN2 is less successful than for TN1.

<u>Additional Treatments.</u>

Some people treat trigeminal neuralgia with complementary therapies, usually combined with drug therapy. These treatments have varying success rates. Complementary treatments for TN include e.g

- Care of some spines mostly in cervical regions.
- Botulinum toxin injections to block sensory nerve activity
- Creative visualization

<u>Application Of DMSO in Treating Trigeminal Neuralgia.</u>

Though not yet approved by the FDA the application of DMSO on the side of trigeminal pain in liquid form can reduce pain or make it bearable, Note; it is from research carried out that the above conclusion where made.

CHAPTER SIX

SCLERODERMA.

What is Scleroderma:

Scleroderma is an autoimmune disease that causes inflammation and fibrosis (thickening) of the skin and other areas of the body. When the immune response tricks the tissues into thinking they are injured, it causes inflammation and the body produces too much collagen, causing scleroderma.

Too much collagen in your skin and other tissues causes tight, hard areas of skin. Scleroderma can affect many systems in your body.

Kinds Of Scleroderma.

Localized scleroderma mainly affects your skin. It has two forms:

- **Morphea:** This means hard oval spots on your skin. They start red or purple and then turn white in the middle. It is prone to affect most functioning organs mostly internal and blood vessels. This is called a generalized morphea.

- **Linear:** This causes thickened skin lines or streaks on your arms, legs or face.

Systemic Scleroderma: also called generalized scleroderma, can affect many parts of the body or systems. They are of two types:

Limited Scleroderma: It appears slowly and affects the skin of the face, hands and feet. It can also damage your lungs, intestines, or oesophagus, the tube that carries food from your mouth to your stomach. It is sometimes called CREST syndrome after its five common symptoms:

- **Raynaud's phenomenon**: This is caused by a lack of blood supply to parts of the body such as the fingers, toes or nose, usually due to cold. Your skin may turn red, white or blue.
- **Calcinosis**: In this case, calcium salts form nodules under the skin or in the organs.
- **Oesophageal dysfunction:** This is when your oesophagus is not working as it should.

- **<u>Sclerodactyl:</u>** This is a thickening of the skin. It usually causes problems moving the fingers and toes.
- **<u>Telangiectasia:</u>** In this case, small blood vessels grow close to the surface of the skin

Diffuse scleroderma: It happens fast. The skin on the middle of the body, thighs, arms, hands and feet may thicken. This form also affects internal organs such as the heart, lungs, kidneys and digestive tract.

<u>Causes of Scleroderma.</u>

Doctors do not know what causes scleroderma. It is one of a group of autoimmune diseases. They occur when your immune system, which normally protects you from germs, instead causes inflammation in your skin and other organs.

<u>Risk factor of Scleroderma.</u>

Anyone can get scleroderma. It usually occurs in women and people between 35 and 55 years of age. some factors capable of increasing risk may include:

- Autoimmune diseases in the family
- Some changes in your genes
- Environmental triggers such as viruses, drugs or chemicals

Scleroderma Symptoms.

- Cuts or sores on fingertips
- Hardened or thickened skin that looks shiny and smooth. It occurs most often on the hands and face.
- Hard, oval spots on your skin
- Painful or swollen joints
- Swelling, mainly in the hands and fingers (oedema)
- Weight loss for no apparent reason
- Difficulty swallowing

Diagnosis Of Scleroderma.

On visitation to a medical professional, he checks you Physically and obtains knowledge of your medical history thus far. They may order tests, including:

- Blood test
- Gastrointestinal tests

- Pulmonary function tests
- Imaging tests such as X-rays and CT scans

<u>Scleroderma Complications.</u>

- Treatment can help reduce the risk of complications, which may include:
- Kidney failure
- Infections
- Scar tissue in your lungs
- Reduction in movement in arms and legs
- High blood pressure in your lungs

<u>Scleroderma Treatment.</u>

You can treat the symptoms of scleroderma by:

- Using recommended anti-inflammatory medications such as aspirin reduces pains and swelling regions Medicines that open the blood vessels in your lungs or prevent tissue scarring
- Steroids and other drugs that slow down your immune system. They can help with muscles, joints or internal organs

- Medicines that increase blood circulation in the fingers
- Blood pressure medications

DMSO Application In Treating Scleroderma.

The DMSO is not officially approved by the FDA as treatment of scleroderma but analysis carried out explained that the scleroderma symptoms remain as Nineteen patients with systemic scleroderma and five patients with localized scleroderma were treated with topical dimethyl sulfoxide using dye and dip techniques.

Partial control was obtained using a very low concentration (5%) on the other side when the contribution was symmetrical.

The duration of the treatment was 3-15 months. Topical dimethyl sulfoxide did not improve skin oedema, range of motion, or Raynaud's phenomenon in patients with scleroderma. No significant beneficial effect on ischemic ulcer healing was observed, and continuous use of dimethyl sulfoxide did not prevent new ulcer formation.

Pain relief was observed in 10 of 16 patients, probably due to the local analgesic effect of dimethyl sulfoxide.

In general, DMSO as seen from the experiment only reduces pain as a result of its applications or administration.

Precaution In Using DMSO For Scleroderma.

DMSO is not currently approved by the FDA to treat scleroderma, it only reduces the pains associated with it.

CHAPTER SEVEN.

Uses And Effectiveness.

Effective On:

Inflammation of the bladder (interstitial cystitis). An FDA-approved medication called DMSO is used to treat interstitial cystitis, a bladder ailment. Using DMSO to wash the bladder can relieve Pain interstitial cystitis symptoms including the discomfort.

Most Effective On:

Brought on by a syndrome known as complicated regional pain syndrome. Empirical evidence indicates that putting DMSO 50% cream on the skin helps individuals with complicated regional pain syndrome feel less discomfort.

- Damage to skin and tissue resulting from chemotherapy leakage from intravenous injection. Certain chemotherapy medications have the potential to damage skin and adjacent tissue if they seep into the skin or surrounding tissue from the vein. If this occurs, research indicates that

- Tendolo: Research shows that DMSO applied topically, along with the drug idoxuridine, reduces the damage and swelling associated with shingles.

Some Ineffectiveness:

A skin disease known as scleroderma. According to the majority of research, DMSO applied topically does not appear to be effective in treating scleroderma patients' symptoms.

Cancer

According to research, DMSO applied topically does not aid in the treatment of cancer.

<u>Other Uses of DMSO Based on Research.</u>

- A disease is known as amyloidosis. Early studies indicate that DMSO may be used to treat amyloidosis by topical application, oral administration, or bladder cleaning.
- Bile canal calculi. According to preliminary studies, DMSO may aid in the dissolution of bile duct stones when combined with specific other solutions.
- Pain relating to cancer. According to preliminary studies, giving intravenous (IV) injections of DMSO and sodium bicarbonate may help persons with cancer-related discomfort feel better about themselves.
- Diabetes-related foot ulcers. According to preliminary studies, patients with diabetes may experience faster healing of their foot ulcers if they apply DMSO to the damaged skin.
- Heightened cerebral blood pressure. There is evidence to support the theory that intravenous (IV) injections of DMSO could reduce hypertension within the brain.

- Inflammation: According to preliminary studies, DMSO applied topically may help lessen osteoarthritis or rheumatoid arthritis (RA) symptoms.
- Gastric ulcers. According to preliminary studies, patients with ulcers brought on by the Helicobacter pylori bacteria or those whose ulcers have not healed after trying various treatments may find that DMSO is a more successful treatment for their ulcers than cimetidine.
- Pressure sores. According to preliminary studies, massaging residents at assisted living facilities with DMSO 5% cream does not help prevent pressure ulcers.
- Promoting skin healing following surgery. According to preliminary studies, topical DMSO treatment may promote wound healing following surgery.
- Damage to the tendon (tendinopathy). According to preliminary studies, patients with tendon injuries may have less pain and improved joint movement after using DMSO 10% gel topically.

- Headaches.
- Gall stones.
- Eye problems.
- Muscle problems.
- Skin problems such as calluses.
- Asthma
- Other conditions

Side Effects In Using DMSO.

DMSO taken as directed by a doctor is LIKELY SAFE. Use only products that your healthcare provider has prescribed. Some non-prescription DMSO products may be "industrial grade," meaning they are not meant for human usage, which raises concerns. These goods MAY BE UNSAFARILY UNSAFE due to the possibility of contaminants that could be harmful to health. To exacerbate the situation, DMSO easily permeates the skin, allowing harmful pollutants to enter the body quickly.

When DMSO is used orally or applied topically, some adverse effects include allergic reactions, dry skin, headaches, nausea, vomiting, diarrhoea, constipation, difficulty in breathing difficulties, visual or eye problems, blood and clotting disorders, and dizziness/drowsiness. Additives such as DMSO also give off a taste and odour similar to garlic.

<u>Safety Special Precautions.</u>

Pregnancy and nursing: The safety of using DMSO while pregnant or nursing has not been thoroughly studied or supported by credible sources. Remain cautious and refrain from using.

- Certain blood conditions. Intravenous (IV) DMSO injections may degrade red blood cells. Those who suffer from specific blood problems may find this.
- Diabetes: Topical administration of DMSO has been reported to alter the body's use of insulin. If you use DMSO in addition to insulin to treat diabetes, monitor your blood sugar levels carefully.

sometimes a method of adjusting insulin therapy can be considered. General Topic.Skin application.

• 77-90% DMSO is usually administered every 3-8 hours for 10-14 days under the supervision of a physician to prevent some of the negative effects of cancer treatment.

• Herpes zoster: Administer 5-40% idoxuridine in DMSO four times a day for four days beginning 48 hours after rash.

• 50% DMSO solution has been used to treat nerve pain for up to three weeks four times a day.

• Osteoarthritis was treated with 25% DMSO gel three times a day and 45.5% DMSO topical solution four times a day.

• Drink a teaspoon of DMSO mixed with water daily to reduce trigeminal pain.

Key Note: It's crucial to remember that applying DMSO topically **MAY NOT BE SAFE**. There have been stories of the self-treatment of several medical ailments with industrial-grade DMSO. Since industrial-grade DMSO may contain contaminants, it is not as high-quality as DMSO utilized in drug research. DMSO readily permeates the skin, carrying with it contaminants and other potentially harmful compounds.

Inside The Bladder.

Healthcare professionals use a tube known as a catheter to drip a DMSO solution into the bladder in cases of chronic inflammatory bladder illness and frequent urges to urinate (interstitial cystitis). After the catheter is taken out, the patient is instructed to wait before peeing to hold the solution.

THE END.